$\mathscr{B}$irth *without*
$\mathscr{V}$iolence

Birth *without* Violence

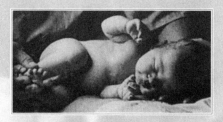

FRÉDÉRICK LEBOYER, M.D.

New Translation by
Yvonne Fitzgerald and the Author

Healing Arts Press
Rochester, Vermont • Toronto, Canada

Healing Arts Press
One Park Street
Rochester, Vermont 05767
www.HealingArtsPress.com

Healing Arts Press is a division of Inner Traditions International

Originally published in France as *Pour Une Naissance Sans Violence* by Éditions du Seuil,
    Paris
First Healing Arts Press edition published in 1995
Revised edition published in 2002
Third edition published in 2009

All the photographs were taken by Frédérick Leboyer and Pierre Marie Goulet except for
those on page 13, 15, and 27, which were supplied by I.M.S. Stockholm.

Note to the reader: *This book is intended as an informational guide. The remedies, approaches,
and techniques described herein are meant to supplement, and not to be a substitute for, professional
medical care or treatment. They should not be used to treat a serious ailment without prior
consultation with a qualified health care professional.*

Library of Congress Cataloging-in-Publication Data

Leboyer, Frédérick.
  [Pour une naissance sans violence. English]
  Birth without violence / Frédérick Leboyer ; new translation by the author and
Yvonne Fitzgerald. — 3rd ed.
     p. cm.
  ISBN 978-1-59477-297-9 (pbk.)
  1. Childbirth. 2. Natural childbirth. I. Title.
  RG661.L3913 2009
  618.4—dc22

                                                                          2009001028

Printed and bound in the United States by P. A. Hutchison

10   9   8   7   6   5   4   3   2   1

Text design and layout by Virginia Scott Bowman
This book was typeset in Goudy Oldstyle

Acknowledgments

I wish to express my gratitude to Yvonne Fitzgerald.
If it had not been for her deep understanding of babies,
her determination, her enthusiasm, and her love of English,
this new translation would never have been written.
And since I feel that all I had been trying to say about
the great mystery that is birth has at last been
fully understood and expressed in an English that is
both literary and poetical,
let me thank her in the name of all mothers and, hopefully,
all the doctors and midwives
who, once they have become aware of the ordeal it is to be born
will meet the young newcomer with more sensitivity, more
intelligence, and more respect.

FRÉDÉRICK LEBOYER

Foreword

Yvonne Fitzgerald

It is hard to remember the stormy, passionate reactions this
book aroused when it was first published in 1974.
While it was greeted with enthusiasm by mothers all over
the world, it gave rise to an outcry in all quarters of the
medical establishment.
And then, little by little, it all cooled down.

Was the message heard and accepted?
I am not sure.
What was a strong wine became slowly watered down into
the kind of herb tea that gives you a good sleep.
And sad, not to say embarrassing, was that this book that
had been written as a tragedy was to be found sandwiched
between brown rice recipes and diapers under the misleading
heading of "childcare."
The kind of misinterpretation that makes people say:
"*Birth without Violence?* It's not a book I would read; I'm
not expecting a baby."

Or

"Latin? Why should I learn Latin? I'm not going to be a priest."
Or else

"*Hamlet?* Why would I read *Hamlet?* I am American; I am not Danish."
Of course the blanket of childcare is more comforting, sounds nicer.
For, after all, who wants to plumb the depths of one's own mind and memory? Who wants to awaken the ghosts lying dormant at the bottom of the unconscious?
Isn't it easier to do aerobics than go through the pangs of psychoanalysis? And it takes the daring of a hero, an Odysseus, to go down into the inferno.

But then, coming back to this book, if it is not just a nice new technique for childbirth, what is it all about?
A story of life and death.
Death! But I thought we were talking about birth.
Who ever suspected that birth and death could be so close?
That it is one and the same door we pass through whether we are entering or taking our leave.
But then, all this is rather frightening.
Frightening? Yes, it is terrifying.
And one could say that the main character in this tragedy is FEAR.
Fear and the child are born together.

And when it dawns on us that this fear of death, which casts such a long shadow over our lives, is nothing but the unconscious memory of the indescribable panic and terror

we experienced when we were born, we begin to see that
there is more to it than meets the eye.

And then we start dreaming.
If this fear could be pacified, healed, the moment we are
born, what an extraordinary life would wait for us.
Too good to be true.
Only when it is seen in this light does this book take on its
true dimension.
Perhaps it is madly ambitious.
Human beings born with this fabulous boon: complete
fearlessness.
Blessed with a life free from anger and aggressivity.
Able to tread the path of life with an unshakable smile and
eyes glowing with burning love.

Because the first translator had not fully grasped the
depths of the message, whole passages, even an entire
chapter, which the translator took to be unnecessary, disappeared.
This is why a new translation was needed, that would give
it back its original flavor, even its disturbing power.
But that needed a new writer.
Because of my great love of English and intuitive knowledge of
the mysteries of childbirth, I was able, working in close
collaboration with the author,
to offer a new translation.
Actually it is not a new or better translation, it is a new book.
As if the text had been born afresh.
With all the literary poetical quality that is necessary
when one tries to tell of the secrets of life, and gives us a

glimpse of its deep mysteries.

The description of a technique was much easier, and would have been an easier way to please a lot of people.

But . . .

There is no such thing as a technique for life.

⁂

From the first time I read this book and even to the present day, it has always been with me.

Over the years I would pick it up again and again and each time discover something new, something I hadn't been able to see or understand earlier, and as I myself progressed through life, so did my understanding of this book deepen. All through these years I always felt that the English version did not do the book justice, especially when I read and began to know the original French edition.

With this in mind, and since the book had sadly disappeared from most bookshops, I proposed to Frédérick Leboyer that we should make a new translation together—he with his deep knowledge of what he wanted to say, and I with my love of English and all my experience from the story of my own birth and the birth of my two children.

Frédérick Leboyer spoke as someone who had once been the baby in this book. On my side, I too have been the baby in this book, but years later came another knowledge of birth. On the day that I gave birth myself I had the feeling that it was "I" who was being born as well as the baby.

Slowly it dawned on me that to be born and to give birth are one and the same; that the very act of giving birth takes a woman back to the moment of her own birth.

This new perception of time, of finding oneself outside the limits of time as we know it, can be very confusing. One becomes aware that giving birth takes place in an altered state of consciousness.

Birth, death, dying, being born or giving birth—nearly all merge at times, all become the same adventure into and out of that territory we might call no-man's-land.

Because this book throws light onto all these mysteries, it remains for me a classic.

Like any mystical text, or as in the practice of martial arts, the further you go yourself, the more layers and levels you uncover, and the more you come to know yourself, the more this book will come and meet you and the more it will give you.

As an Homage

to the Talent and Wisdom
of the Co-translator

Dear Yvonne,

What am I to say about your foreword?

Simply that it is great.

In just a few pages you've said, about the mysteries of Birth

as much, if not even more than what my text is telling.

How was that possible?

Very simple!

Being Irish, you are a born writer, a born poet,

as well as a perfect mother.

Once again, to you, all my admiration

as well as respect.

FRÉDÉRICK LEBOYER

Part One

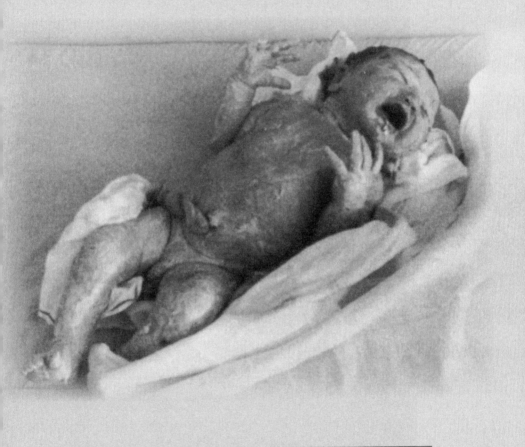

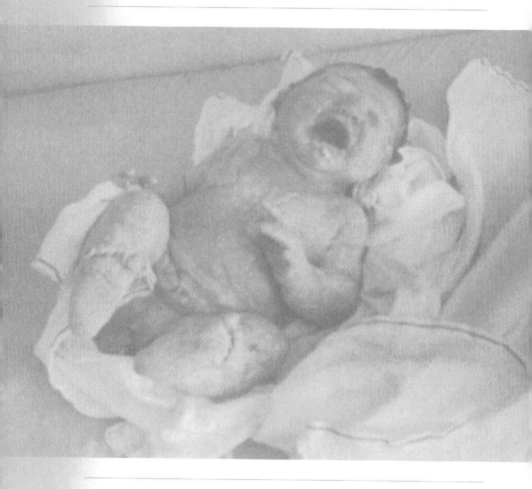

"To be born is to suffer."

—GAUTAMA

1

Do you think babies enjoy being born?

What do you mean, enjoy being born?

Exactly what I said. Do you think that birth is a pleasant experience for the child? That this newcomer is happy to have entered our world, find itself being in our company?

Happy . . . Neither happy nor unhappy, since a newborn does not feel anything.

Is this what you think? And how do you know?

Well, it's obvious. Everyone will tell you.

That's not much of a reason.

But at this age. And when it is still so small.

As if size could have anything to do with feeling, with pain! How can an intelligent man like you talk like that?

Well, I must say . . .

So, for you, the newborn does not feel pain?

No, he does not.

Then how is it that he cries? And cries so bitterly?

Must be very stupid as well. Have you ever heard a newborn cry?

Yes, I have. And, true, it breaks the heart. You may have a point. Although . . . how could he, since he doesn't yet have consciousness?

No consciousness? You mean he has no soul?

No, no. I don't mean a soul. I don't know anything
about the soul.

But consciousness? Yes, about consciousness, yes,
you know? Wonderful! At last I've found someone who
can explain this great mystery, My friend, I am on
my knees! At your knees! Tell me, please, do let
me know what consciousness can be!

Well . . . you see . . . consciousness . . . in fact . . .

2

Let's not continue this discussion.

Arguing is refusing to see things as they are.

Things, that is to say, facts.

The simple fact is that as soon as a child is
born he starts to cry, and how bitterly.

And although this is very strange, it is the one
thing that delights everyone there.

"How beautifully my child cries!"
exclaims the happy mother, thrilled and amazed that
something so little can make so much noise.

Does this crying simply mean that all the reflexes
are normal and that the machine works?

So man is nothing but a machine?

Or could the cries be trying to express some pain,
some terrible sorrow.

If the baby is crying with such intensity, doesn't it
mean that he's suffering terribly?

Could childbirth be as distressing for the child as
for the mother?

And if so, does anyone care?

It doesn't seem so, judging by the way we treat
the new arrival.

Alas, it seems a deeply rooted idea that "it"
doesn't see anything, "it" doesn't hear anything.
How, then, could "it" feel anything like sorrow
or pain?
The answer is simple:
"it" cries, "it" screams,
in short,
"it"
is an object.

And what if, by any chance,
"it"
is already
a person?

3

The newborn baby . . . a person?

Now, really.

Medical books will tell you quite the opposite.

Books . . .

How often does the scientific truth of one day become
the lie of the next?

So how do we know what is what?

Looking at the facts,

that is to say, asking the person concerned, the
child, might give us the answer.

The trouble is that a newborn baby can't speak.

And yet when you think of all the noise he makes,
it's hard to say he cannot express himself.

If a Chinese man breaks his leg, although you may not
speak a word of Chinese, you can understand his
screaming perfectly.

And when it comes to screaming, who in the world
can scream like a newborn baby?

And if you won't take my word for it,
see for yourself.

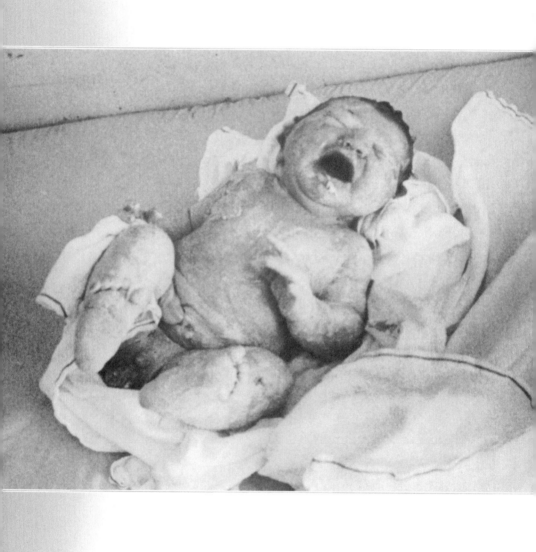

4

What else is there to say?
The tragic forehead, the screaming mouth, these
closed eyes, clenched eyebrows, these desperate,
pleading, outstretched hands, these feet,
furiously kicking, the legs curled up to protect
the tender stomach, this flesh, which is nothing but
a mass of spasms, jolts . . .
How could you say that a baby doesn't speak when
with his whole being he's protesting:
"Don't touch me! Don't touch me! Leave me
alone!"
And at the same time begging:
"Help me! Somebody please help me!"

Has there ever been such despair in one voice?
This child is in agony.
But nobody even hears it.
Isn't that extraordinary?

5

"Do you mean to say that . . . the reason this baby is
crying so bitterly . . . do you think he's trying to
tell us . . ."
"Your mind will use any trick in order to block out
what it really means to be born.
Looking at the pictures we've seen, people might say:
'But that's not a normal birth. This baby is being
tortured by sadists!'
Sadists?
No.
Just ordinary people like you and me.
And if you don't believe me,
just look. Just see."

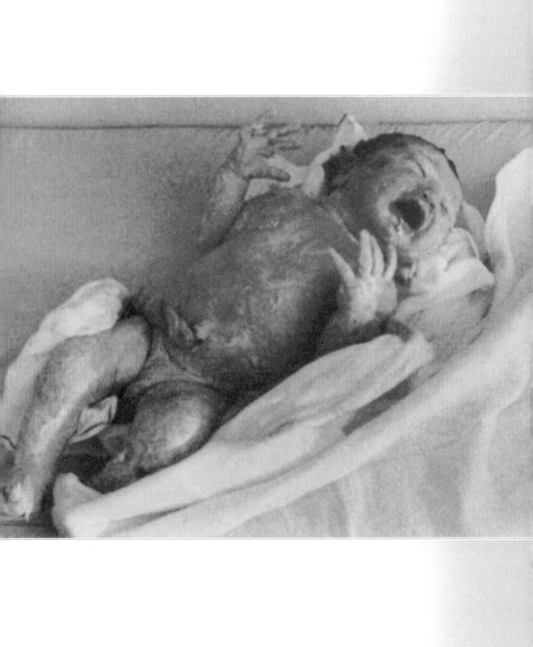

6

The Holy Family.

In its modern version, that is.

A child has just been born. The mother and father look on delightedly. Even the young obstetrician smiles. The same look of wonder and happiness lights up all their faces.

Everyone is radiant with happiness.

Everyone except the child.

The child?

You hadn't even noticed the child, had you?

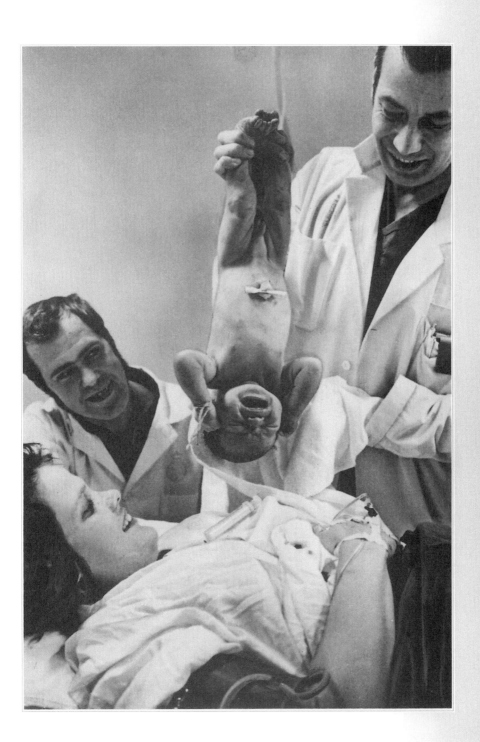

Oh no! This can't be true!
This mask of indescribable agony, these hands
clutching, clinging onto this head, like someone
struck by lightning, shattered, who at any moment
is going to fall to the ground, like a mortally
wounded soldier.

This . . . a birth?
It's a murder.

And in the midst of all this suffering,
the parents . . . in rapture!

But it can't be true!
No! It can't be true!
And yet, it is true.
Yes, this is birth

for the child.

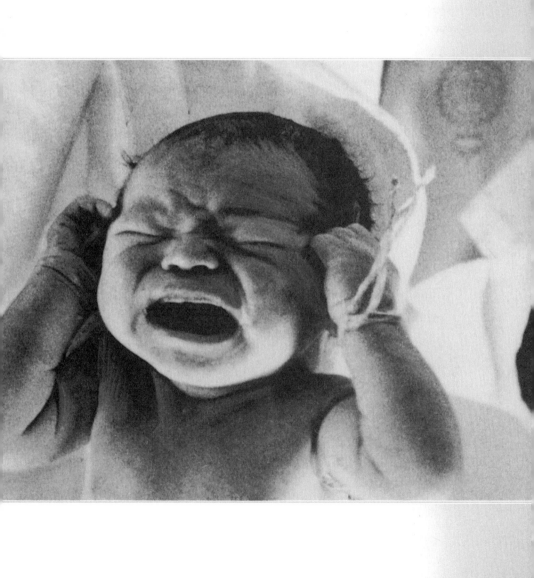

7

Isn't it amazing how blind we can be?

Let us try to understand why.

Actually it is simple.

Take the young doctor; what is he smiling about?

The happy child?

Not exactly.

"His" delivery has been a success. Mother and baby

are doing well, so this man is pleased.

Pleased with himself, that is to say.

And the mother?

Blissfully happy as she smiles at her baby.

Maybe she's smiling because it's over.

She's done it!

She's very relieved, and more than anything, she's

proud.

Proud of herself most probably.

The father?

This man, who has more than likely never done very much

out of the ordinary, has managed to produce

(or so he is thinking!) a son and heir!

A small heir who's going to carry on the accomplishments

of his parents!

Of course he's proud!

In fact, you could say everyone is delighted.

All delighted with themselves,

except . . .

the child.

8

Isn't it a tragedy?

We should be crying tears of shame, crying for our own
blindness.

The same blindness that made us think women had to
suffer simply because we didn't know any better.

Happily we no longer believe in the old saying:

"In pain shall ye give birth."

Isn't it time to do for the child what we've been
trying to do for the mother?

9

But what can be done for this poor child?

Are we to look to the amazing advances in modern
technology for the answer?

No. Quite the contrary.

It was only when we asked what causes a woman to suffer
when she gives birth that we began to see it was
her FEAR that made her fight and tighten up, lock
herself into the vicious circle:

the more pain, the more fear,

the more fear, the more pain.

With the same simple approach let's try to
understand what makes the child suffer.

Part Two

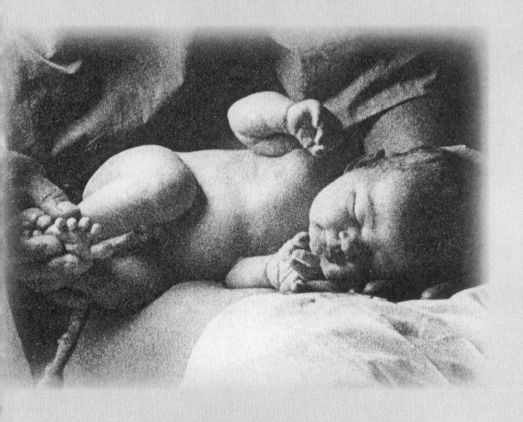

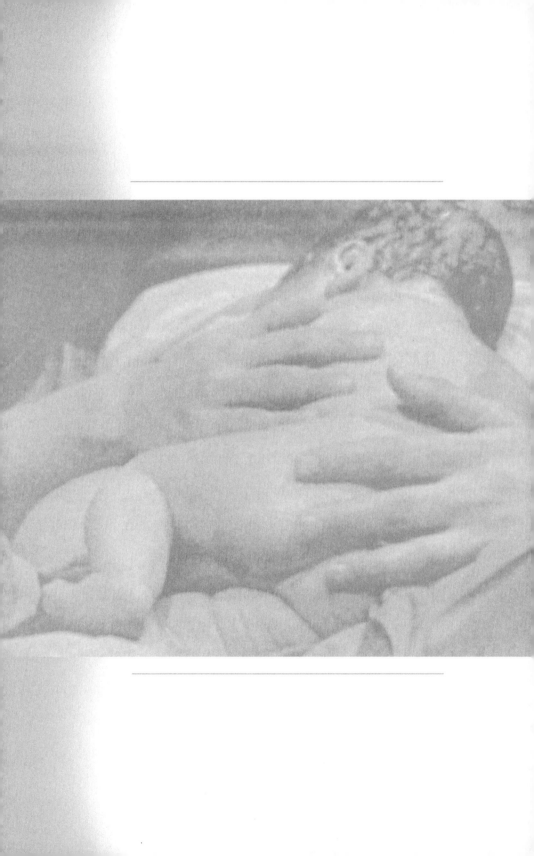

1

To be born is to suffer.

Birth is pain.

For the woman, as we all know, and for the child,
as we have forgotten.

Now that we are finally aware of it, let us try to
understand why.

What is it that makes being born such a horror?

2

The nightmare of being born is not so
much the pain as the fear.

For the baby, the world is a terrifying place.

It is the vastness, the enormity of the whole
experience of being born, that so terrifies this little traveler.

Blindly, madly, we assume that the newborn baby feels
nothing.

In fact, he feels . . . everything.

Everything, totally, completely, utterly,
and with a sensitivity we can't even begin to
imagine.

Birth is a tempest, a tidal wave of sensations
and he doesn't know what to make of them.

Sensations are felt more acutely, more strongly by the child,
because they are all new, and because his skin is
so fresh, so tender,
while our blunted, deadened senses have
become indifferent.

The result of age, or maybe of habit.

3

Let's begin with sight.

A newborn baby cannot see.

Or so we are told in books, and have come to believe.

Otherwise, we could never

shine a light straight into the eyes of a newborn baby

as we do.

What if we were to lower the lights as the child is being

born?

But why lower lights for someone who

is blind?

Blind?

Maybe it is time that

we

opened our eyes.

If we did, what might we see?

Just as the head emerges, while the body is still

prisoner, the child opens his eyes wide. Only to

close them again instantly, screaming, a look of

indescribable suffering on his tiny

face.

Are we trying to brand our children with the marks of

suffering, of violence

by blinding them as we do with dazzling lights?

What goes on before a bullfight?

How is a furious charging bull produced, mad with

pain and rage?

He is locked up in the pitch dark for a week
then chased out into the blinding light of the arena.
Of course he charges! He's got to kill!
Perhaps there lurks a murderer in the heart of
every man as well. Is it surprising?

4

Now hearing.
Do you imagine a newborn child is deaf?
No more than he's blind.
By the time he arrives in this world he's been
aware of sound for a long time. He already
knows many sounds from the universe that is his mother's
body:
intestines rumbling, joints cracking,
and that spellbinding rhythm, the heartbeat;
even nobler, grander,
the throbbing undercurrent, the swell,
sometimes the storm
that is "her" breath.
Then . . . "her" voice, unique in
its quality, its mood, its accent, its inflections.
Out of all of which is woven, as it were, this child.
From a great distance come the sounds of the
outside world.
What a symphony!

But remember that all these sounds are muffled,
filtered, cushioned by the waters.
So that once the child is out of the water, how the
world roars!
Voices, cries, any small sounds in the room
are like a thousand thunderclaps to the unhappy
child!
It is only because we are unaware, or because we have
forgotten how acute the sensitivity of a newborn baby is
that we dare talk at the top of our voices or even, at times,
shout out orders in a delivery room.

Where we should be as spontaneously and respectfully
silent as we are in a forest or a church.

5

Now we begin to suspect what a calamity,
what a disaster it can be to be born,
to arrive suddenly into the midst of all this
ignorance, all this unintentional cruelty.
What about the newborn baby's skin?
This timorous skin that quivers at the slightest
touch, this skin that knows if what approaches is
friend or foe and can start to tremble,
this skin, raw as an open wound, which until this moment
has known nothing but the caress of the friendly
waves lapping it.

What is in store for it now?
Roughness, insensitivity,
the macabre deadness of surgical gloves,
the coldness of aluminum surfaces,
the towels, stiff with starch.
So the newborn baby screams,
and we
laugh delightedly.

6

Once the scales begin to fall from our eyes
and we become aware
of the torture we've made of birth,
something in us cannot but shout
"Stop! Just stop!"

Hell is no abstraction.
It exists.
Not as a possibility in some other world at
the end of our days,
but here and now, right at the start.
Who would be surprised to learn that such visions
of horror haunt us for the rest of our days?

Is that it, then?
Is that the extent of the torture?
No.

There is fire, which burns the skin, scalds the eyes,
engulfs the whole being, as if this poor baby had
to swallow this fire.
Think back to your first cigarette, or your
first whiskey, and remember the tears it brought
to your eyes, how your choking breath protested.
Such a memory might begin to help you understand how
the baby feels drawing in his first gulp of air.
Of course the baby screams, his whole being
struggling to expel this vicious fire,
to fight bitterly this precious air, which is
the very substance of life!

So it all begins with a "NO!"
to life itself

7

If even that were the end of the suffering,
the pain.
But it isn't.
No sooner is the child born than we grasp his feet
and dangle him upside down in midair!
To get a sense of the unbearable
vertigo the child experiences, we must go
back a bit, back to the womb.

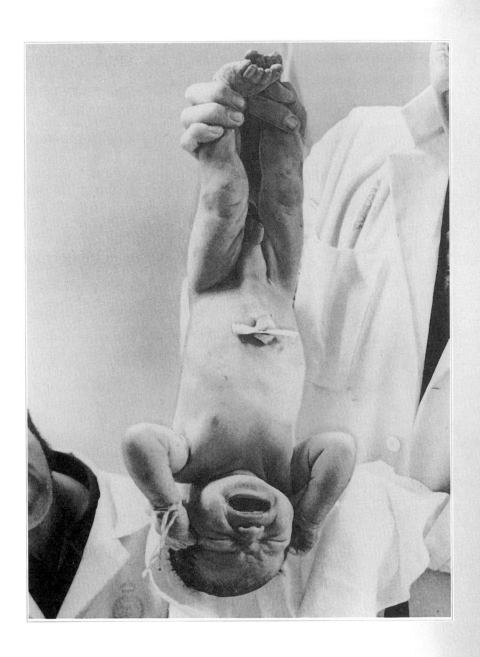

8

In the womb the child's life unfolded like
a play in two acts;
two seasons, as different as summer from
winter.
In the beginning, the "golden age."
The embryo, a tiny plant, budding, growing,
and one day becoming a fetus.
From vegetable to animal; movement appears,
spreading from the little trunk outward, to the extremities.
The little plant has learned to move its branches,
the fetus is now enjoying his limbs.
Heavenly freedom!
Yes, this is the golden age!
This little being is weightless; free of all shackles,
all worries.

Carried weightless by the waters,
he plays,
he frolics,
he gambols,

light as a bird,
flashing as quickly, as brilliantly as a fish.

In his limitless kingdom,
in his boundless freedom,
as if, passing through the immensity of time,
he tries on all the robes,
he tastes and enjoys all the forms
that Life has dreamed up for itself.

Alas, why must it be that everything must become
its own opposite?
This is, unfortunately,
the Law
to which all things must bow.
So it is that, dancing in tune to this Universal
Breath,
Night leads toward Day,
Spring to Winter.
It is the inevitable law that turns the enchanted
garden where the child once played so freely
into a garden of shadows and sorrow.

During the first half of pregnancy the egg
(that is to say the membranes that surround and contain
the fetus, and the waters in which he swims) has
been growing more quickly than the child.
But from now on the reverse becomes true:
the fetus is now growing much bigger, becoming
a little child.
The egg does the opposite. It has achieved its own
perfection and hardly grows anymore.

Because he is growing so large, one day the child
comes upon something solid—the walls of the uterus—
and learns for the first time that his kingdom has
boundaries.
Because he keeps on growing, the space around him
becomes more and more confined.
His world seems to be closing in on him,
gripping him in its clutches.
The former absolute monarch must now reckon with the
law!
Careless freedom, golden hours!
My foolish youth!
Where have you gone?
Why have you left me?

The child, once his own master, now becomes a
prisoner.
Immured.
And what a prison.
Not only do the walls press in on him,
squashing him from all sides,
but the floor is coming up to meet him,
even as the ceiling is descending slowly,
relentlessly, forcing his neck to bend.
What is there for him to do but bow his head in submission,
accept this abasement?
And wait.

9

But one day he is rewarded for his
humility.
To his surprise the grip is now an embrace.
The walls are suddenly alive, and the clutch has become
a caress!
What's happening?
His fear is changing into pleasure!
Now he revels in the very sensations that first made
him tremble.
When they come he quivers with pleasure,
curves his back,

bends his head

and waits,

but this time with anticipation, with wonder.

What is happening? . . .

What is the reason for all this?

Contractions.

The contractions of the final month of pregnancy,

warming the uterus, preparing it for its new role.

But then one day . . .

the gentle waves lash into a storm . . .

and there is anger in this embrace!

It's grinding, crushing, instead of holding,

cherishing!

The once pleasant game has become horrible. . . .

It's not being caressed, it's being hunted.

I thought you loved me,

but now you're squeezing me, killing me,

pushing me down.

You want me to die,

to launch myself into . . . this emptiness,

this bottomless pit!

With all the strength he can muster,

the child resists.

Not to leave, not to go, not to jump . . .
anything . . . but not this void.
He's fighting not to be cast out, not to be expelled,
and of course he's going to lose.

His back stiffens, his head hunches down
into his shoulders,
his heart thumps as if it will break, the child
is nothing but a mass of terror.
The walls are closing in on him like a
winepress crushing grapes.
His prison has become
a passageway,
which is turning into a funnel.

As for his terror, which is limitless,
it has turned into rage.
Animated by rage,
he's going to attack.
These walls are trying to kill me,
they must give way!
And these walls are . . .
my mother!
My mother who carried me,
who loved me!

Has she gone mad?
Or have I?
This monster won't let go.
My head, oh, my poor head,
this poor head that bears the brunt
of all this misery.
It's going to explode.

The end is in sight.
It must mean death.
How can he know, this poor, unhappy child,
that the darker the gloom, the obscurity,
the closer he is to reaching
the light, the very light of life!

10

It is then that everything seems to
become chaos!
The walls have released me, the prison, the dungeon
has vanished.
Nothing!
Has the entire universe exploded?
No.
I am born . . .
and around me,
the void.

Freedom, unbearable freedom.
Before, everything was crushing me, killing me, but at
least I had shape, I had some form!
Prison, I cursed you!
Mother, oh, my mother, where are you?
Without you, where am I?
If you are gone
I no longer exist.
Come back, come back to me,
Hold me! Crush me!
So that I may be!

11

Fear always strikes from behind.
The enemy always attacks you from the rear.
The child is wild with anxiety
for the simple reason that he is not being held
anymore.
His back, which has been curled up for months,
which the contractions have drawn taut as a bow,
is suddenly released,
like a bow having let fly its arrow.
But what a shock!
To calm, reassure, and pacify the
terrified child, we must gather up his little body,
hold it back from the void, save it from this unwanted

liberty, which he cannot yet taste or enjoy,

because it came all at once, and far too quickly.

We must help him the same way we regulate the air
pressure

for a deep sea diver who has surfaced too fast.

What fools we are!

Instead of gathering up the little body,

we hang it by its feet, leaving it swinging in the void.

As for the head, this poor head,

which has borne the brunt of the catastrophe,

we let it dangle, and give the poor child the sense

that everything is whirling, spinning,

that the universe holds nothing but unbearable vertigo.

12

Next, where do we put this martyr, this child

who comes from the security, the warmth of the womb?

We put him onto

the freezing harshness of the scales!

Steel, hard and cold, cold as ice,

cold that burns like fire.

A sadist couldn't do better.

The baby screams louder and louder.

Yet everyone else is in rapture.

"Listen! Listen to him cry!" they say,

delighted at all the noise he's making.

Then he's off again.

Carried by his heels of course.

Another trip, more vertigo.

He's put somewhere on a table and we abandon him, but not
for long.

Now for the drops.

It wasn't enough to stab his eyes with light
directed right onto his face, now we've got something
even worse in store for him.

Since we are the adults, we are the stronger,
we decide . . .

13

Of course, we prevail.

We force the tender eyelids open,
to apply a few drops of burning liquid. . . .

Drops.

Drops of fire, supposed to protect him from an
infection long since eradicated.

As if he knows what's coming,
he struggles like one possessed,
he squeezes his eyelids tightly together
trying desperately to protect himself.

14

Then he's left on his own.
Adrift in this incomprehensible, insane, hostile
world,
which seems bent on destroying him.
Escape! Escape!
Suddenly an amazing thing happens:
at the limit of his tears, the limit of his breath,
to escape.
Not that his legs can take him anywhere, but
he can flee to within himself.
Arms and legs clasped, curled up into a ball,
almost as though he were a fetus again.
He has rejected his birth, and the world as well.
He's back in paradise,
willing prisoner in a symbolic womb.

15

But his precious moments of peace don't last
long.
He must be elegant, reflect well on his mother!
So for her sake he is squeezed into those implements of
torture we call clothes.

16

The glass has been drained to its dregs.
The worn-out, defeated child gives up.
He lets himself fall back into the arms of his only
friend,
his one refuge:
sleep.

17

This torture, this slaughter of an innocent,
this murder
is what we have made of birth.
But how naive, how innocent to imagine
no trace will remain;
that one could emerge unscathed, unmarked, from
such an experience.
The scars are everywhere:
in our flesh, our bones, our backs,
our nightmares, our madness,
and all the insanity, the folly of this world—
its tortures, its wars, its prisons.

Of what else do all our myths and legends cry,
all our holy scriptures,
if not of this tragic odyssey.

Part Three

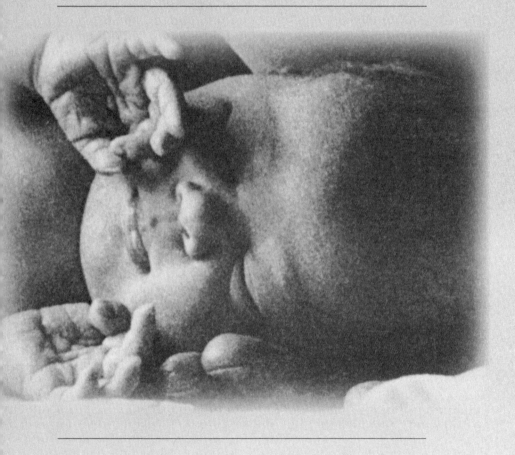

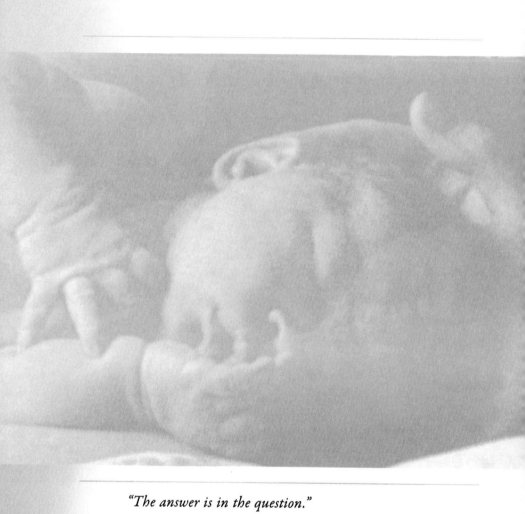

"The answer is in the question."

1

We were wondering about how best to prepare the
child . . .
Now we can see it's not the child who needs
to be prepared.
It is ourselves.
It is our eyes that need to open,
our blindness that has to stop.
If we used just a little intelligence,
how simple things could be.

2

In short, everything begins in paradox.
The child was in prison,
and as soon as he's free,
he yells.
This, they say, often happens to prisoners.
We open the cell doors
and the freedom makes the prisoners disoriented,
goes to their heads!
In fact, they begin to behave as if they missed
their cells, their jail, and would prefer to be locked up
again!
And unconsciously they do everything they
can to find themselves once more safely behind bars!

In the same way, seeing the newborn baby panic-stricken
by his freedom, you feel like saying:
"Why are you crying?
You are absolutely miserable when you should be
rejoicing!
Try to understand what's happened
so you can enjoy your new freedom!
See how you can stretch yourself,
play, and move around!
What are you crying about?"

At that point everything seems to be in a state of
complete confusion, almost impossible to repair.
And yet it is all very simple.
As we shall see.

To communicate we must speak to the child in a language
he can understand, one that doesn't rely on words
and yet may be understood by anyone.
Love.
Speak . . . the language of love . . . to a newborn!
Why, yes, of course!
How else do lovers communicate?
They don't say anything, they simply touch.
Because they are modest and shy, they shun the
light,
prefer darkness, night.

In obscurity, in silence, they
reach for each other, wrapping their arms around
each other, they re-create the old prison
in which they feel safe, protected
from the world outside.
Their hands speak,
and it is their bodies that understand.

So this is the way to talk to the newborn:
in silence and darkness,
with gentle and loving hands,
that reassure and move slowly,
and in time with his breathing.

But let us go step by step,
sense by sense, as it were.

3

Let us begin with sight.
Like lovers, let's turn down the lights.
Who could make love under a spotlight?
Therefore let's keep only the least light—a candle
for instance—for the sake of the doctor's vision.
How peaceful, how calming this half-light is,
and so much in keeping with the mother's own inner
silence.

4

Now hearing.

Nothing could be simpler; all we have to do is

remain silent.

Simple?

Perhaps it's not as easy as it sounds at first.

The mind is so noisy.

It is not always easy to stay silent in the company

of others.

One has a tendency to think of something and feel impelled

to say it.

Yet it is only if we pay attention to the other,

and to our own depths, that we will experience that

something beyond words.

But silence is not something that comes spontaneously

to us, rather we must search for this and call it up

from deep within us.

In fact, the first women who experienced

silence in childbirth found it so new that they were

disturbed, even frightened.

As the end of labor is approaching, there should be

very few words spoken in the room.

In the quiet you can feel that you are coming
very close to something of gravity.
The silence will be like the hush that settles over the room
of someone who is dying.
Perhaps it is the same threshold we cross,
whether coming or going.

Such an almost tangible silence has a most powerful
effect on the child, although how or why cannot
be explained.
Yet it dispels the panic,
holds back the fear that was waiting to
surge up within the child.
Of course, at times it is necessary to say something,
to give an instruction.
This must be whispered, almost
inaudible.
When we first attempted this,
our hushed voices took women so completely by
surprise that they were overtaken
by panic. In this intense
silence all the mothers could hear . . . was that
they couldn't hear anything!
The children responded spontaneously to
this tranquillity.

But the mothers' eyes, as they darted from one
face to another, begging for an answer,
told of the women's surprise.
Unable to hold back, they burst out:
"Why isn't my baby crying?"
It was agonizing.
It was astounding. It was heartbreaking.
"Why isn't my baby crying?"
It was like the cry of an inconsolable child whose toy was
not what he had been hoping for.

We had not thought it necessary to tell the
mothers beforehand that their babies probably would
not cry.
And because this silence seemed so pleasing to us,
it had never occurred to us that it might frighten
the mothers.
But "My child isn't alive!" would wail the despairing
voice.
It was ludicrous.
"Your child is fine!" we would whisper.
The whispering made things worse.
"What are you whispering about? Is my baby dead?

Oh no! My baby is dead!"
Dead! Even as the child was wriggling and moving
on her belly.
"Stop!" we would say. "Dead people don't move!
Can't you feel your child moving; can't you sense
How happy he is?"
But our words went unheard.

All this made us realize that we should have
explained to the mother what was going to
happen. A silent, happy newborn is so
new and unexpected, it goes completely
against accepted ideas.

So we tried, although a bit late, to explain
the silence: that it was maintained out of
respect for the child, out of concern for his ears,
that we were quiet because we didn't want to frighten
him with our loud voices. We tried to explain to the
mothers that it is no more necessary for her child to
be born suffering and screaming than it is that
she go through hell in order to give birth.
Our explanations came too late. Their eyes remained
full of doubt, of regret!

5

This education, this initiation into silence is
just as necessary for all those who
attend the woman when she's giving birth: the
obstetrician, the midwife, the nurses.
People tend to speak loudly in delivery rooms,
often shouting their words of encouragement:
"Come on, push! Push!"
Which is a complete mistake.
Intended as encouragement, these loud exhortations
are instead most disturbing
for the mother.
For a woman in labor is in
what might be called an altered state of
consciousness, and hypersensitive to
the slightest noise or movement around her.

6

Darkness, or almost, and . . . silence.
A profound peace settles in the room.
You can feel the respect that naturally
attends the arrival of a baby.
One doesn't shout in a church.
One spontaneously lowers one's voice.

If there is such a thing as a sanctified place, surely
it is the room the child is about to enter.

Subdued light, silence . . . what else is needed?
Patience.
Or rather, the sense that one should slow down
and thereby enter into another rhythm; the profound
rhythm of life,
to which the mother has spontaneously become attuned,
and which is also the tempo of the child.

Unless you have re-created this incredible languor
in your own body, it is impossible to understand
birth. Impossible to meet the newborn on his terms.
In order to reach this deep understanding, to arrive at
a place where you can meet the child, you have to, as it
were, step out of time.
Step out of *our* time.
Meaning our strong, familiar sense
of how time is flowing, of the apparent speed with which,
for us, it seems to flow.
Our sense of time and the time sense of the
newborn baby are practically irreconcilable.
The one is a state of near statis,
the other state, ours, is often a frenzied restlessness,
close to madness.
Besides, we adults are never "here."
We are always somewhere else.

In the past, in our memories.

In the future, in our plans.

We're always looking back, at what is gone,

or ahead, at what is yet to happen.

Never focusing on "here and now!"

Yet if we have any hope of rediscovering the newborn baby,

we must step outside of our own furiously running time.

Which seems impossible.

How can we step out of time?

How can we escape its fast and furious flow?

The only way is by trying to be fully with the present moment.

Yes, to be here *and* now, as if there were no yesterday, no tomorrow.

To allow any thought that the moment

will end, that another appointment awaits,

is enough to break the spell.

As usual, everything is very simple.

And apparently impossible.

How can we reconcile the irreconcilable?

How can finite combine with infinite?

It can only happen if we open completely to the other,

which means completely forgetting oneself.

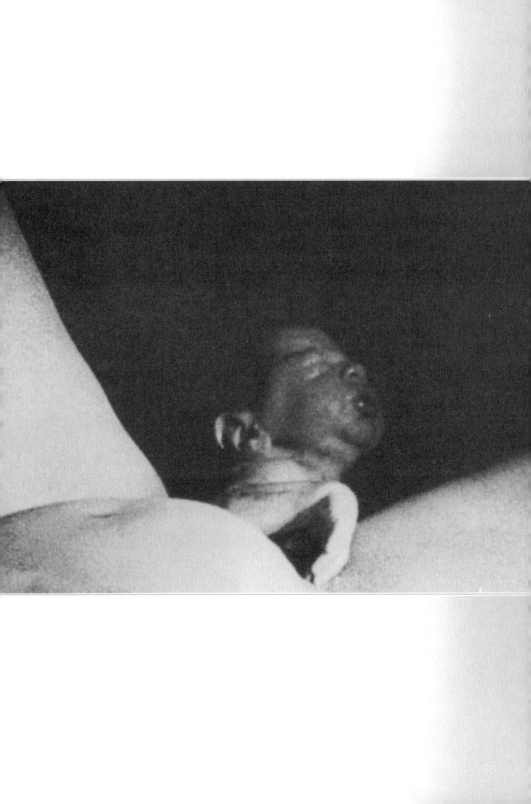

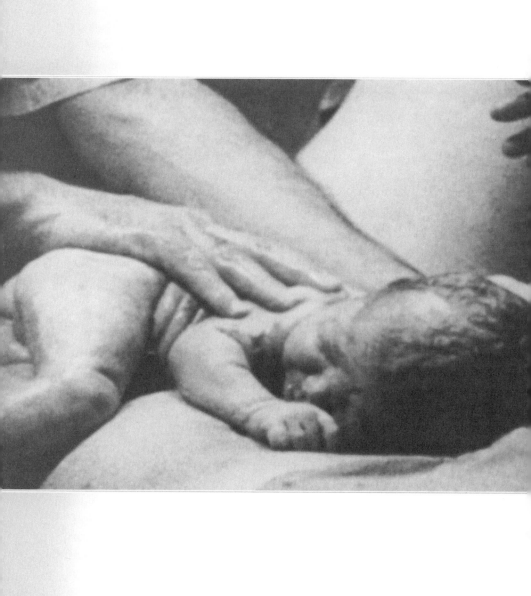

7

Now the stage is set.
The lights are dimmed.
The curtain may rise.
The child can make his entrance.
At last he is here.

8

Head first, and then his shoulders, one after the
other.
Either all this happens naturally, or some help is
needed at this critical moment.
As soon as the head is out the child wants to draw breath,
which is impossible for him because his chest is still
imprisoned in his mother's body.
If the shoulders are stuck, his progress
comes to a halt, and help is needed quickly,
because anguish is building up furiously in
the child.
How can we help?
By sliding a finger under the child's armpit we can help
the rotation of his body and liberate the little prisoner.
Then, holding him under both arms we hoist him
out, as if pulling him from a well, and put him
straight onto his mother's belly.
Most important of all, we never, never, at any time
touch his head.

He's lying on his mother's belly.
And where better to receive the child than this
belly. It has the exact shape to receive
the baby. When he was within, it was rounded and convex;
it has now become hollow, and waits like a nest to cradle
the child.
Soft and supple, it moves with
the rhythm of the mother's breathing,
and the living warmth of her body makes it
the perfect place for the newborn to be.
Finally, and this is most important, because the
baby remains so near to her, the umbilical cord can remain
intact.

9

Cutting the cord the moment a baby has emerged from his
mother's womb is an act of extreme cruelty, and harms
the baby to an extent that is hard to believe.
Leaving it intact, however, so long as it
continues to beat, transforms the whole birth experience.
For one thing, it forces the obstetrician to be
patient, and leads him, as well as the mother, to respect
the rhythm, the sense of time ordained by the child.
Besides, leaving the cord intact allows the
natural physiological changes to take place within the
child's body at their own pace.

We have already described the way air suddenly rushing
into the baby's lungs has the same effect on him
as a burn. But there is more.
Before his birth, the child lived in oneness.
For him there was no difference between
the world and himself, because inside and outside were
one. He knew nothing of polarities. He didn't
know about being cold, for example, because cold
cannot exist without heat. The body temperature of
the mother and the baby are exactly the same. How
then could he appreciate any contrast?

So you might say that before birth, there was neither
inside nor outside, any more than there was hot or
cold.
As he enters this world, the newborn baby encounters
for the first time a kingdom of opposites in which
everything is either good or bad, pleasant or
unpleasant, agreeable or disagreeable, wet or dry.
What is the gate through which he enters this kingdom
of opposites?
Not through his senses, that comes much later,
but through breathing.
When he takes his first breath, he crosses a threshold,
a border.

He breathes in, and from this action is born its
opposite: he breathes out.
And then in turn . . .

Thus he is launched irrevocably into the eternal
cycle, the never-ending oscillation, the very principle
of our world, in which everything comes back to this
breath, this pulsation.
He is in the world where everything, for always,
is born of its own opposite:
day from night, summer from winter,
riches from poverty, strength from weakness,
never ending,
without beginning.

10

To breathe is to become one with the world outside,
to tune in to the music of the spheres.
Its function is to make the blood take in oxygen
and get rid of wastes, mostly carbon dioxide.
But in this simple exchange, two worlds come
near each other, try to mix and touch: the world
of outside and the world of inside.
Two worlds, separated, try to reunite:
the interior world of the organism, the little "I,"
and the exterior world, the vast universe.

It is in the lungs where they meet—the blood
mounting from one's own depths, the air
coming from above.
The blood and air rush to conjoin, anxious
to mix and mingle.
Of course they can't, separated as they are by
the barrier of the alveol membrane.
Both sigh for this lost oneness.

The blood arrives in the lungs, depleted of its
oxygen, its strength spent, dark with waste: the carbon
dioxide, which makes it old.
Here it is going to rid itself of its old age, gain its
energy, rejuvenate.
Transformed by this visit to the fountain of youth, it
departs, alive, red, and rich!
It returns to the depths where it gives forth its riches.
Once more lets itself be filled with
wastes, and then returns to the lungs. Thus the cycle
continues indefinitely.
As for the heart, it keeps pumping, pushing the blood,
sending it, rich and red toward the thirsty tissues of
the organism, and sending it back when it has
become old and worn-out, for renewal to
the lungs.

How does all this happen in the fetus,
where the lungs are not yet working? The blood of
the fetus, just like ours, needs to be renewed.
The placenta fulfills this role.
Among other things it does, it takes the place
of the lungs.
The blood comes and goes through the umbilical cord,
which contains three conduits, a vein and two arteries,
covered by a sheath.
So the blood of the fetus renews itself not by contact
with air in its lungs, but in the placenta by contact with
the blood of the mother, which in her lungs . . . and so on.

The mother, in effect, breathes for the baby, just as
she eats for him, carries him, protects him, sleeps and
dreams . . .
Yes. The child is completely dependent
before his birth.
But then what happens?
A total upheaval: The blood that until then flowed
through the cord suddenly rushes into the lungs!
The child abandons the old route, he leaves the way of
the mother.
In the act of drawing breath, of oxygenating his own blood
with his own lungs, the child becomes himself, in effect
saying, "Woman, what do we have in common?
I no longer need an intermediary between myself and the
world."

Of course it is only a first step, for all the rest he
still relies totally on his mother.
But it's a step in the right direction.
With his first breath, the child sets forth on the road to
independence, to autonomy, to freedom.
But practically speaking, much depends on the way
this transition takes place.
Whether this transition is made slowly, progressively, or
brutally, in panic and terror, can make the difference
between a gentle birth
. . . or a tragedy.

11

If the changeover comes abruptly it will leave a mark
for the rest of life. Any future change will always be
perceived as threatening.
Of course, the child must not, at all costs, be deprived
of oxygen, not even for one moment.
Here there is no quarrel with medical science,
which agrees perfectly with nature's plan.
Nature provides oxygen for the
child through two sources:
the cord continues to beat, even as the lungs begin to
function.
The two systems work together, one taking over from the
other, like a relay. The first, the cord, continues
to oxygenate the child until the new system, the lungs,
has taken over completely.

Although the child is out of the womb, he remains dependent on his mother through the umbilical cord, which continues to beat strongly for several minutes, four or five,
sometimes even longer.
Oxygenated through the cord, and thus protected from anoxia, the child can, without shock or danger, settle down to breathing without being rushed, in his own time.

12

What should we do during these critical few minutes of the transition of the blood from the old route through the placenta to the newly working lungs?
We must understand that Nature herself doesn't take sudden leaps and has her own pace. She has left this time, these few minutes, so that this changeover from one world to another can be made with ease.
She has made it so that the baby is oxygenated from two sources for several minutes as, at the same time, an orifice in the heart closes, and the baby is then safely on his own.
For a few minutes the baby straddles two worlds, as it were. Then slowly, slowly he can cross the threshold from one to the other peacefully and easily, and with all safety,

as long as we don't rush in, interfere,
and can manage to quell our old reflexes, our nervousness,
born, in fact, out of the anxiety of our own birth.
The effect on the well-being of the child will be
immeasurable.

We are all so quick to blame Nature, when actually
she's so full of love and wisdom, and it is only we
who are too blind to see.

Whether the cord is cut abruptly or allowed to stop
beating of its own accord completely changes,
even determines the way in which a child perceives his entry
into the world, and, consequently, the way he will react
to the continuous change that is life. You might say
that his perception of this moment will color the rest
of his life.

If we cut the cord immediately, we create a situation
that is the opposite of the one Nature intended.
By clamping the cord before the lungs are fully operative
we deprive the child's brain of oxygen.
The organism cannot but react violently to our aggression,
and then a whole system of stress comes into play.
Not only will we have done something absurd and

uncalled for, but we will have set up what Pavlov called a
conditioned reflex, which will recur
throughout life.
What have we linked together?
Life and breath,
breath and the fear of impending death.

What geniuses we are!

13

You might then ask, How is it that, even when the
transition has been allowed to take place in its own
time, the child may still give a cry or two?
The answer is simple.
The thoracic cage, now that nothing is compressing it,
suddenly expands, thus creating a void.
The air rushes in and it burns.
Naturally the child tries furiously to expel the air.
This is the first cry.
Then, often, everything stops.
The child pauses, as if dumbfounded by his own suffering.
It can happen that he might repeat the cry two or three
times before this pause.
Then when this pause comes, it is we who
panic. And usually . . . a slap on the bottom
follows. But now that we know better and can control

our impulses, our fears, and trusting the strong beat of
the cord, we can keep our hands to ourselves.
Soon we will see . . .
breathing beginning again of its own accord.
Hesitant at first, timid, careful, it will still pause from
time to time, marking little breaks.
The child, oxygenated as he is by the cord, is pacing himself
and taking in only as much of the burning element
as he can put up with, then pausing, only to start again.
As he gets used to it, he begins to breathe more deeply.

14

Soon he learns to enjoy what, in the beginning, was so
very painful. Very soon his breathing, which was
at first so hesitant and doubtful, becomes joyous.
In all, the child has given only one or two cries.
All we hear now is a deeply peaceful breathing,
punctuated by short cries, exclamations of surprise,
or even sighs of pleasure.
Mixed with this breath are the sounds the baby
is making with his lips, his nose, his throat.
A language all his own.
And never, never, those screams of terror,
those wails of despair, those hysterical shrieks.
Maybe a child has to give one or two cries when he's
being born,

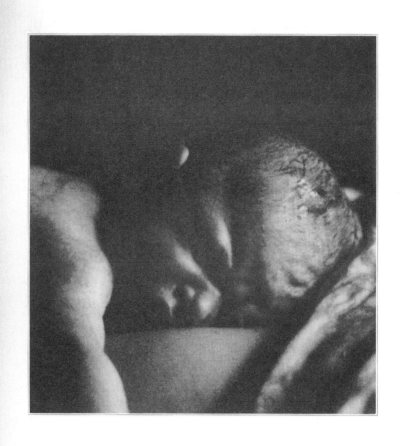

but must they be cries of anguish?
Because the child is pleased with this new experience,
tasting it in all its newness, he can easily forget the
world he has left behind.
No regrets, not a backward glance.
Coming into life is like waking from a long and pleasurable
sleep, and not from a nightmare.
When the present is so delightful, why cling to the past?

Now that the cord has stopped beating, we can cut it.
Not a sound, no crying, no cause for alarm, not even a
tremor; it has simply become obsolete, and so can be
removed.
An old bond has been left behind.
We have not wrenched the child from his mother;
they have simply parted, and will go their separate ways.
Why would the young traveler yearn for the past
when his voyage ends so happily and he has found the other
bank, so tranquilly, so surely?

How intelligent, what a blessing such a birth is.
Because we left the cord beating it is as if
his mother had accompanied him across the border, and led
him gently into this formidable and forbidding world.
Just as later, when he learns to walk, she will be there
offering him her hand to hold.

An open hand that the child can grasp and let go of as
he takes his first tentative steps.
What a poor mother it would be who suddenly
withdrew her hand the moment her child began to trust his
own strength.

15

Learn to respect this sacred moment of birth,
as fragile, as fleeting, as elusive as dawn.
The child is there, hesitant, tentative,
unsure which way he's about to go.
He stands between two worlds.

For heaven's sake, don't touch him,
don't push him,
unless you want him to fall.
Let him wait until he feels
the time is right.

Have you ever watched a bird take flight?
As he's still walking, he's heavy, awkward,
his wings drag, and then suddenly
he's flying,
graceful, elegant and free.
He was the son of earth,
now he's the child of the skies.

Can you say when he left one kingdom for the other?
It is so subtle, the eye can hardly catch it.
As subtle as stepping in,
or out, of time,
to be born,
or to die.

What of the tide
that imperceptibly,
irresistibly rises,
only to fall?
At what moment did it turn?
Is your ear sharp enough to hear the ocean breathe?

Yes, this birth,
this wave parted from wave,
born from the sea
without ever leaving her.
Don't ever touch it with your rough hands.
You understand nothing of its mysteries.
But the child,
the drop from this ocean,
knows.

A wave pushes him toward the shore,
another pulls him back,
only to push him higher still.
One more
and he's out of the flood.
He's parted from water
and come to the land.
He's frightened, terrified.
Let him be.
Just wait.
This child is awakening
for the very first time.

This is his first dawn.
Allow him its grandeur, its majesty.
Don't even stir until he leaves behind
the night and its kingdom of dreams.

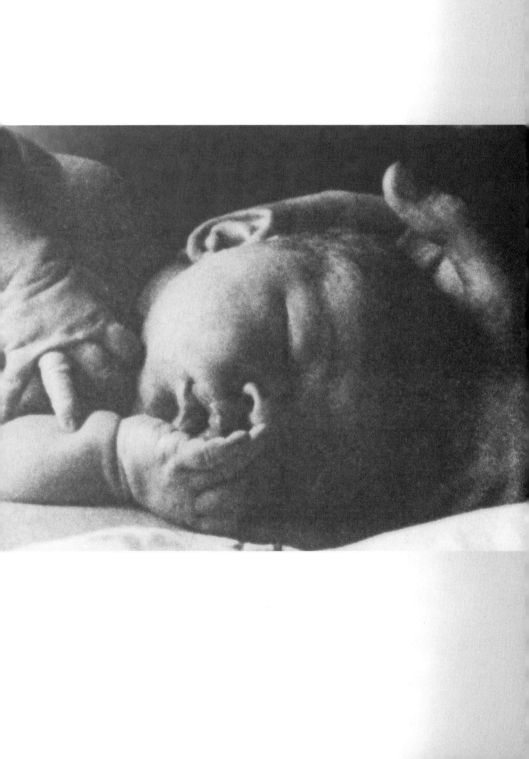

16

The rest, you might say, is detail.
Once breathing is well established, everything is
accomplished.
All has either succeeded or failed.
But details, as always, are not without importance.
For example, in what way should we put the baby on
his mother's belly?
Should we lay him on his side, on his stomach,
or flat on his back?
Never flat on his back.
That would cause the spinal column, which has been
curved for so long, to straighten all at once.
It would suddenly let loose all the dormant energy
locked in there and the shock would be too much. It
would be like an explosion.
Let the child unfold his back when he feels ready
himself.
Don't forget that each child comes equipped with
his own character, his own temperament, his own pace.

There are some who are no sooner born than they lift their
heads proudly, draw themselves up, and stretch out
their arms as if to say:
"I'm here!"

These are the strong ones, who settle into their
new kingdom as if they were kings.
Their spines straighten with the force of a
tightly strung bow releasing its arrow.
But sometimes, the very same children will then
withdraw, pull back, frightened by their own
audacity, their own bravery.
There are others who start off curled up in a little
ball, and only open up little by little, making
their discoveries cautiously.
Because we cannot anticipate what's to come, the best
thing to do is to put the child flat on his belly,
with his arms and legs tucked under him.
This is a familiar posture, the one that
best allows the abdomen to breathe freely and
the baby to work his way, at his own speed, toward
the final unbending.

Then, because the child is on his front,
we can keep an eye on his back, and see how he is
breathing.
In fact, the bending of the spine, of the back, and
the beginning of breathing are all one.
We can watch how breathing takes over the
whole of the baby's body. Not only the chest but
also the belly, and especially the sides.

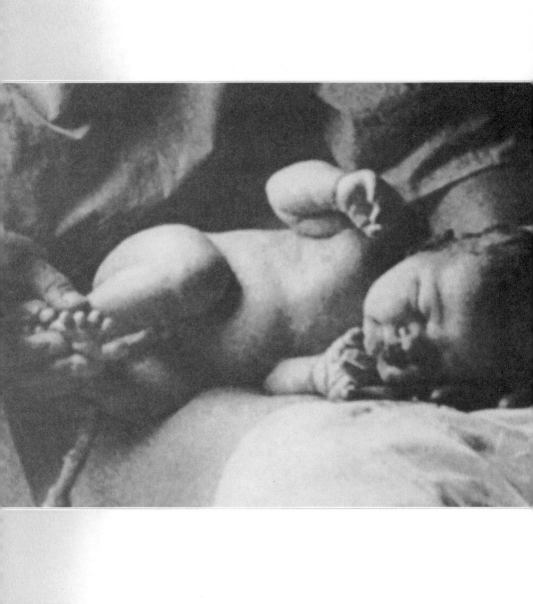

Very soon the baby is nothing but breath,
which passes like a wave from the top of his head
to the small of his back.
This wave is like the shadow of the contractions,
which, like waves themselves, pushed the baby to
the shore.
At the same time it is like watching a tree
start to grow.
Out comes an arm, usually the right, stretching
like the branch of a tree.
Then the other. Both seem surprised that nothing
stops them anymore, that space can be so limitless,
so vast.
It's like watching branches grow out of the power of
the breath. The breath is to the child as the sap is to the
tree.
Now the legs.
One after the other, like roots, which will one day
stabilize this tree. But not yet. For
the time being they are still very tentative, for
they have had to fight their way out of the
enchanted cave.
In order to allay their panic, all that is needed
is to offer them some limit: an open hand the baby's
feet can meet, offering gentle resistance but
able to be pushed away.

Otherwise, the baby will feel completely
disoriented.
So, little by little, everything settles down,
or rather, everything comes together harmoniously.
Soon, just as if he is waking from his first sleep,
the baby stretches out with a complete sense of his own
well-being.
Since, while all this has been happening, the
cord has stopped beating, we are now ready for the
next step. But let us go slowly, pausing often.

17

Haven't we come a long, long way?
We are out of the water, we have touched dry land.
We've left behind the ever-moving, changing, treacherous
kingdom of the fishes.
Now it is the earth that carries us.
Earth, which is steady, tranquil, sound, and true.
Earth we can trust.
For the very first time, nothing moves.
What a surprise.
But since there is a price for everything, we now know
for the first time how it feels to be heavy.
We'll have to crawl.
And yet the skies are there, above our heads.

It is their light, their divine light that gave us
the courage to emerge.
And they will give us the courage to stand and walk.

What a long, long road, this path from mineral
to man.
The path each must tread again when he's
come to taste the joy that is life.

What else are we doing when we pray?
Nothing but returning to the source,
the source of all life,
as if going through the whole adventure again.
Wanting to pay homage to Earth, our mother,
we kneel.
With folded arms and a humble heart
we bow to the ground.
Our forehead touching the dust we say,
"I obey,
for I know that in your wisdom and love
you know better."
There we remain, folded up, empty,
as empty of that precious breath as the child
not yet born who hasn't yet tasted that pleasure of life.

Having paid our respects, expressed our gratitude
to the one who carries us,
to whom we owe everything,
into whose womb we will return at the end of our days,
we arise.

Like a bow
that has let go its arrow,
how vibrant we feel
when, unfolding, we let the air and its joy
fill us full—
as vibrant as we were the day we tasted
our very first dawn.

This, in truth, is prayer.
Since to pray is to be born anew
to the fullness of life.

But then, can one pray in a hurry?
Can it be rushed?
As with the child who's just arrived,
who's joined us,
can't we grant him
a moment of time?

18

A few words about the hands that will hold the newborn
baby.
These hands are the first thing that the child will encounter.
The language they speak is the primal language, the
language of touch.
This is how mother and child were communicating.
It was through the child's back that he
received her messages.
Now that he's born, naked and disoriented,
the way we touch him is crucial.
Most of the time, the hands
of the doctors, the midwives, and the nurses are not gentle
enough.
Simply because they have not realized what it means to
the child.
Because these hands are so unaware, and move much too
quickly, they terrify the child.
Let them be gentle but firm.

Most of all, let them move very, very slowly.
Everything we do for the newborn baby is too rushed, too
hurried for one who is only just entering time.
At this moment, what the child needs is to be massaged,
just as newborn animals need to be licked by their
mothers—the act without which they
often die.

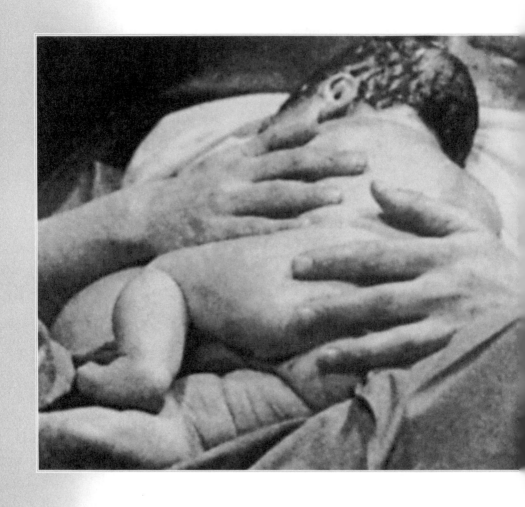

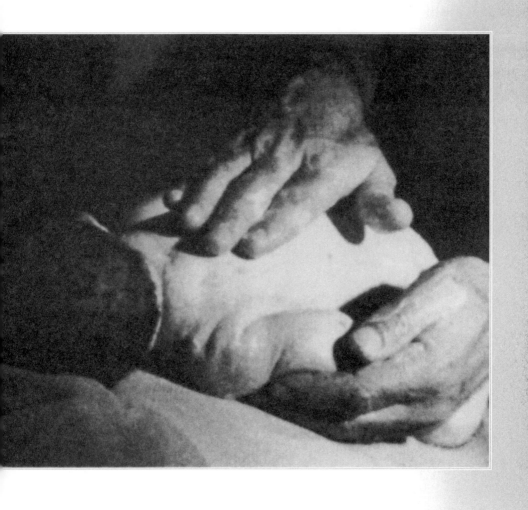

It is most important that the hands that will massage
the baby's back can rediscover the rhythm he knows,
the rhythm of the contractions, the rhythm that moves
with the outward breath.
What the child wants to feel again is not the wild fury,
the storm of labor, but the embracing waves that told him
of his mother's love.
Our hands should travel along his back,
one following the other,
like wave after wave
breaking onto the seashore.
The rhythm of dancers, of lovers.
Love . . . and the child!
Yet what is it lovers are looking for,
if not to heal the rift,
return to the primal sea,
rediscover its infinite pulse?
A return to paradise,
a pilgrimage back to the source.

19

So much for rhythm, for movement.
But there is something else that can be transmitted through
hands, even hands that are not moving.

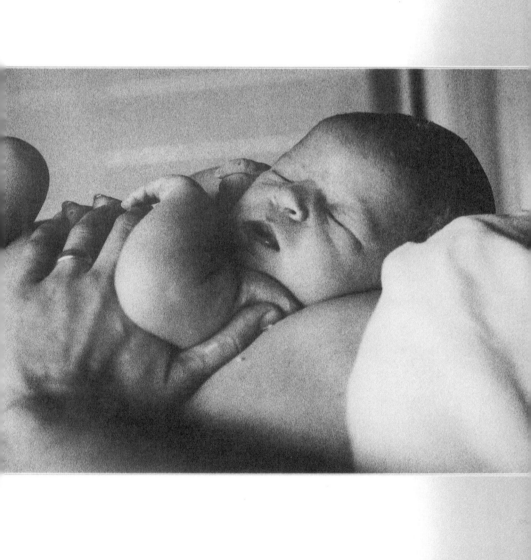

The child is still so sensitive that he will know by
the feel of the hands resting on him whether he is
loved or refused, accepted or simply being carelessly
handled.
Under caring hands, the child opens up and lets go.
Whereas under stiff, mechanical hands, he feels
he's being clutched by claws, and of course
he closes up, withdraws in panic, as if to escape to
within himself for protection.

20

Naturally, it's the mother's hands that should hold
the child.
But often she's still overcome by her own
emotions, her own fears, which she's hardly had
time to leave behind.
Her hands are not yet steady and sure.
If someone else, such as a loving midwife, is
there, calm, and able to transmit her inner peace,
her hands would be better in the beginning, until the
mother has had time to catch her breath.
It's not that we want to take the child away from his
mother, but the intensity of what she's just lived
through can still be affecting her so strongly that it
overwhelms the child.
In these crucial moments, the child needs peace,
quiet, and calm.

Often mothers don't know how to touch their babies.

Or maybe they just don't dare.

Some deep inhibition seems to hold them back, stop them.

Why?

Possibly because the child has just come from a part of the body we don't want to, don't dare to mention.

Perhaps it's our education that makes us step back, as if this part of us does not exist, or at the very least, is not something we talk about.

So the mother finds herself in a troubling, conflict-filled situation, torn between her natural urge and her inhibitions, product of her repressive education.

21

Now let's come back to the child.

The fullness of his breath tells us that all is well.

The cord has been cut.

It is as if centuries have passed and yet it has only actually been a matter of a few minutes.

What comes next?

However blissful this time has been for mother and baby, it must come to an end.

The child cannot stay on his mother's belly all his life.

Just as the child had to depart from the womb, now he
will have to leave his mother's body.

To meet with what?

This first step in life cannot be but terrifying.

How can we ease it and pacify this terror?

In the same way that giving a new toy to a child makes it
easier for him to part with the one he's been playing with,
so we must find a way to make him enjoy his first
moment of separation and thus gladly accept that he's on his
own.

Of course we're not going to put him on
ice-cold weighing scales, and even the softest towel
cannot compare with his mother's body.

What could be the answer?

Water.

This is where he has come from, and what he's known
all his life. It's gentle, it's familiar.

It is this very familiarity that in the end
will completely calm him. It will be like
meeting an old friend when one is far from home.

This feeling of something familiar saves the child
who is lost in an overwhelming world of new sensations.

A bath has been prepared in a small tub, filled with
water at body temperature, or slightly higher since
it's going to cool down quickly.

With the permission of the mother, who must be willing,
we take the child,
and slowly, slowly we ease him into the water, feet
first of course.
A sensitive eye can catch how intense the experience is
for the child.
As soon as he finds himself back in water, he becomes
weightless again.
Water has, as it were, once again taken the load off
his body.
His joy and feeling of relief are hard to describe.
We have nearly accomplished a miracle, we have turned
this first separation, which is always loaded with
anguish, and which shadows us all our life, into a joy.
One can feel any remaining tensions in the baby
melt away, vanish under our hands.

And as these tensions melt away,
and what is left of his fear disappears, and
the child feels so safe, he even dares to open his
eyes.
No words can describe the depths of this first look.
It is as if he is asking all the questions of man
in that single moment.

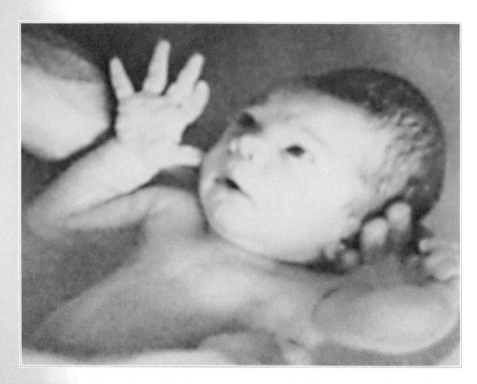

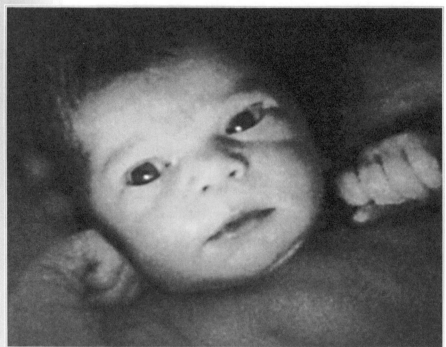

Then it becomes so clear that life does not start now, at
this point, but that the child was aware long before
he came to us, and has merely crossed a threshold.
In disagreement with all classical psychology, anyone
who has witnessed such a birth cannot but
exclaim:
"But this child *is* looking! . . ."
Whether he sees in the way we do is another
issue.
Maybe we have to accept that there are many ways of
seeing, of knowing.

22

Completely free from fear, and his first surprise over,
he begins to explore his kingdom.
His head turns to the left, to the right, as if
enjoying its new freedom.
Out comes one hand from under the water, it opens and
reaches toward the sky.
Then the other.
His hands move in such harmony you'd think you were
watching
a ballet.
They meet, clasp, and part,
moving with all the grace of an underwater plant.
As for the legs, a little hesitant at first, soon they too
begin to stretch and play.

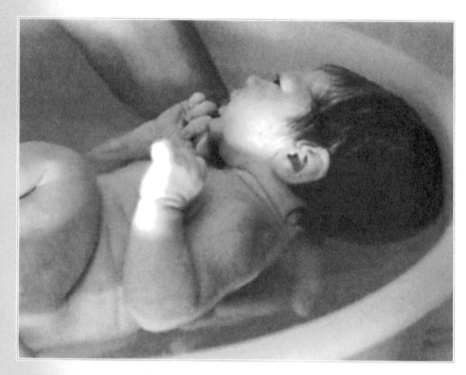

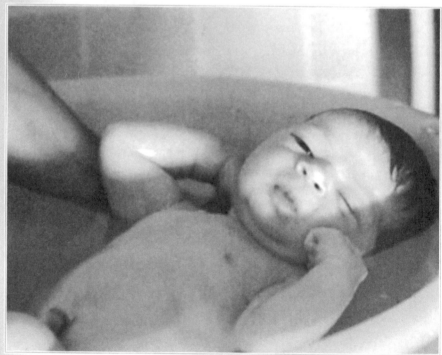

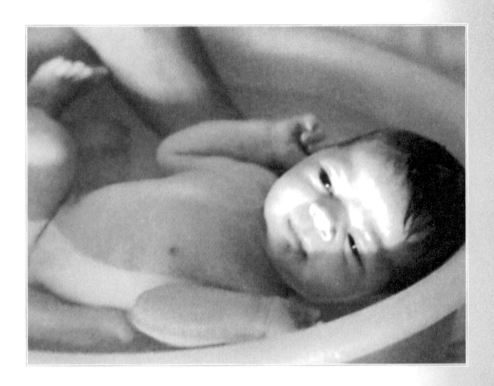

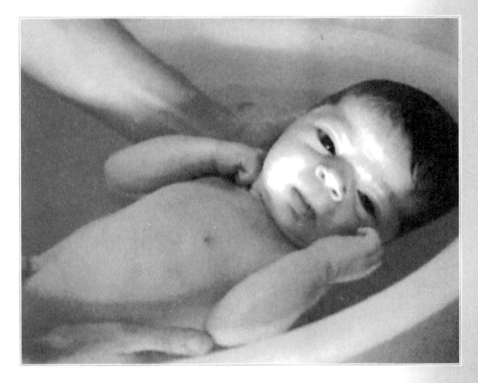

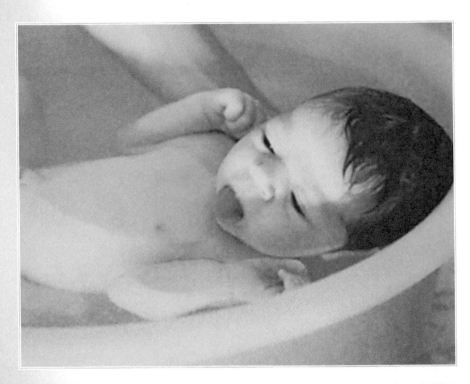

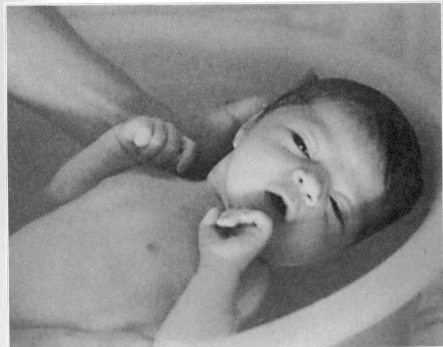

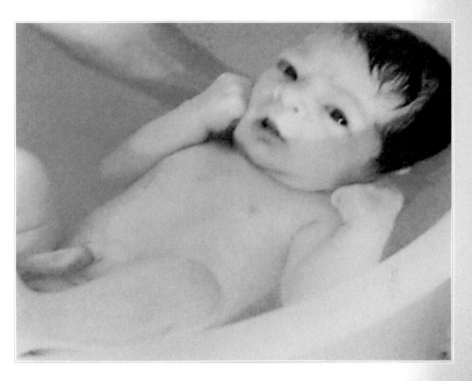

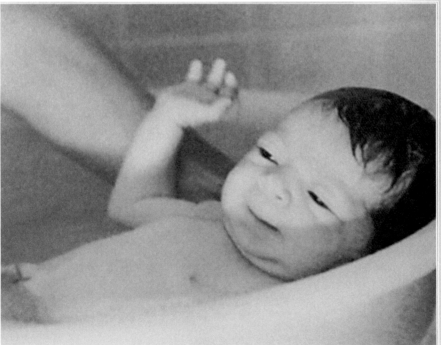

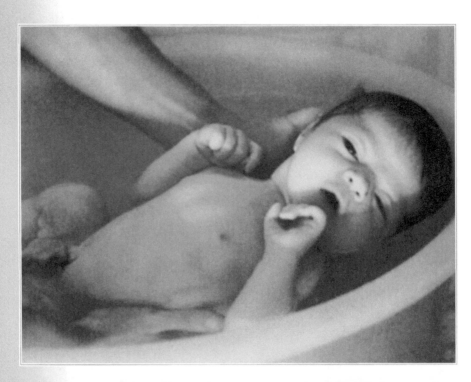

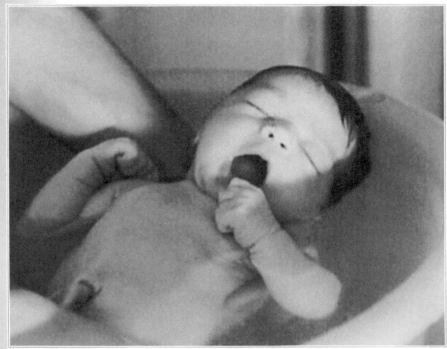

And here it is important to say that the feet of the
baby should always be able to find the edge of the bath,
to find a limit, as it were. Otherwise, if they meet
with nothing, the child will experience the same panic as
a swimmer out of his depth.

Because his first experience has been so
rich and so pleasant, this baby will always be an
adventurer.
Life, for him, will always be a challenge, which he
will meet with confidence and courage and an eagerness
to try to taste everything new that
might cross his path.
Is not the constant newness of life, its continual
change and variety, the thing we find
most difficult?

23

Now that fear has subsided, and been left behind once
and for all, let us try to be free of the past and
its fascination.
Let's try to take the step out of the sea,
to land,
and meet with the earth.

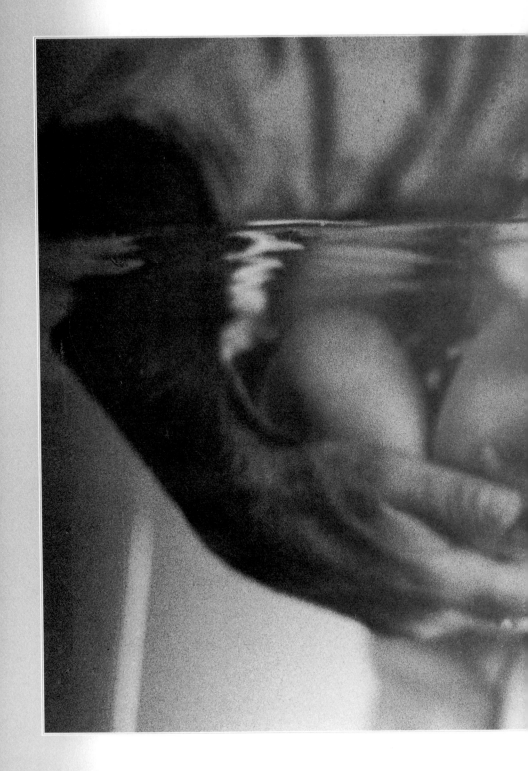

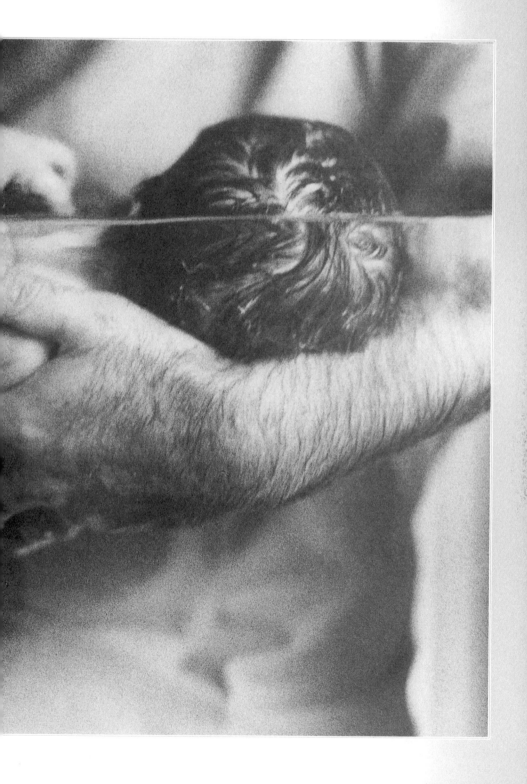

Fourth step.
Fourth station of this calvary that is birth,
where there is neither sin nor punishment.
It is truly an odyssey,
and the hero, the newborn,
has accomplished something so difficult.

So little by little we begin to take the child out
of the water.
If he doesn't like this idea and protests,
because once again he's feeling all his own weight,
we don't force him, but lower him back in again,
only to try to take him out a moment later.
Once again he protests,
goes back to the water,
and comes out again,
and what at first seemed unpleasant
now becomes a game.
This game we play with him,
lifting him out and lowering him back in the water,
is a way of playing with weight and weightlessness.
Isn't it true that no matter the culture,
children all over the world love to
swing,

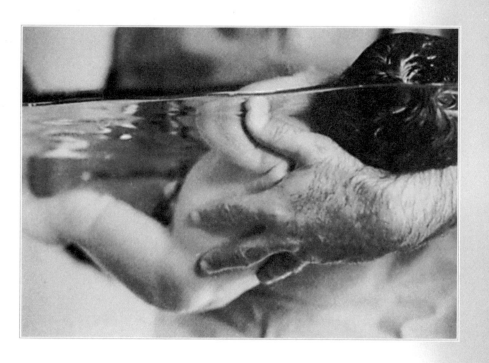

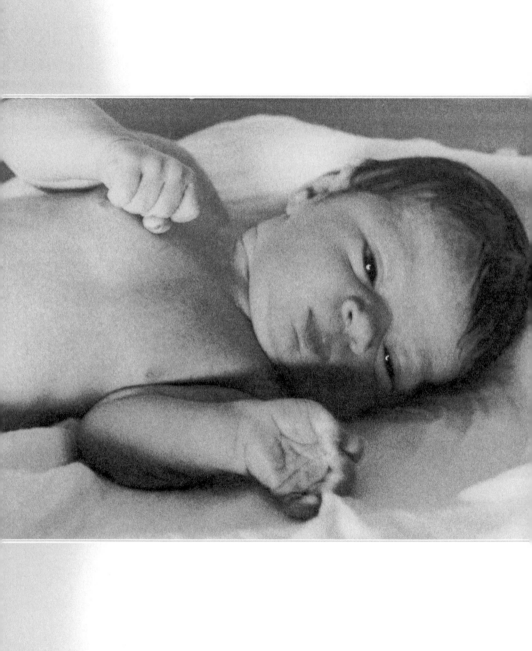

which makes them, in turn, heavy as a stone, and light as
a bird?
Eventually we lift him out completely,
dry him gently, and swaddle him in something warm,
letting him experience for the first time this feeling that
nothing is moving.
Another new and extraordinary feeling for him.

Remember that all those months he spent inside his
mother, everything was moving, whether his mother
was walking or simply breathing quietly in her
sleep.

24

But now, for the first time . . .
and how strange . . .
nothing is moving at all!
This is the majesty of Earth.
For all those children who have been rushed into the
world, who haven't been led gently from water to land,
from movement to stillness, with so much love,
intelligence, and patience, waking up on their own will
always frighten them.
This immobility will always terrify them.
But for the child whose birth has been such a blessing,
these fears will not exist.
He'll be free forever from nightmares and guilt.

25

How impressive it is to watch this child open
his eyes wide, begin to feel his way around,
explore all that surrounds him.
All with no panic, no tears.
On the contrary, with a seriousness, a gravity
that's hard to believe.
Yes, this child is truly like a wise man, an old soul,
because whatever he does, it is with complete
awareness.

But also it seems as if something is emanating
from this child.
He seems to radiate a peace, a serenity, that he's
brought from somewhere far beyond.
The words of Lao-tzu come to mind:

"One who possesses virtue in abundance, the Holy one,
is like a newborn babe."

But what is this "virtue"?
It has nothing to do with morality, being virtuous.
Virtus in Latin means "courage, vitality, virility."
What Japan and China call chi,
and India, Shakti.
It is the secret, silent power of a Zen Master,

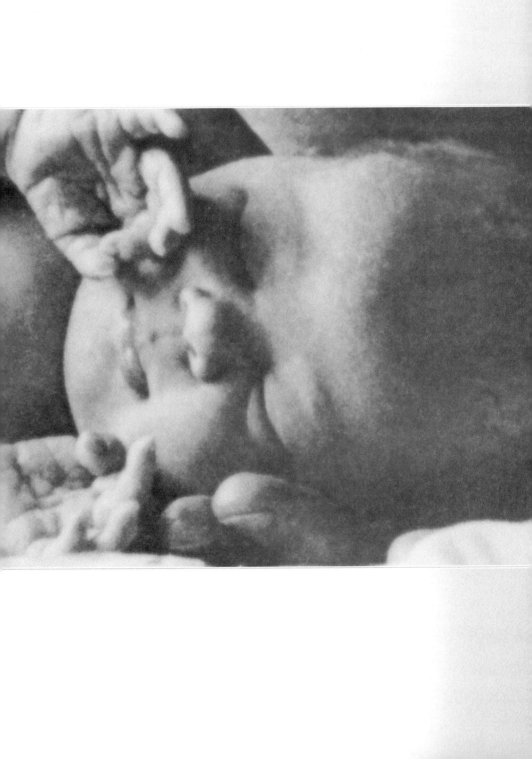

a true Master of Martial Arts,
or a saint.

For one who is sensitive enough to feel it,
sense it,
it is this "virtue,"
this grace,
this chi, this Shakti
that silently flows,
shines like a blessing
from the newborn.

Part Four

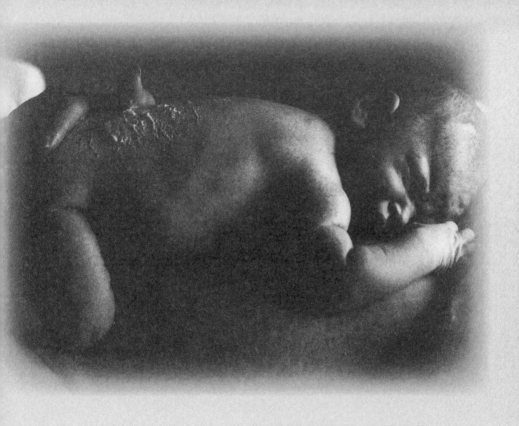

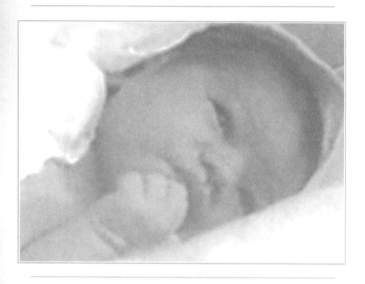

"In the pursuit of learning
one knows more every day.
In the pursuit of the way
one does less every day.
Less and less until
one does nothing at all.
And when one does nothing
there is nothing
that's left undone."

—Tao-te Ching

1

Now our story draws to a close.
Now that the child has tasted the joy of being
on his own and the wonder that is stillness,
let him return to his mother.
Not in a panic, not because he's looking for someone,
anyone to save him, as one might cling to any
branch when drowning, or seek any port in a
storm.
No, it is with eyes wide open, in all awareness
and with inner peace, that these two will meet.
Lying once again on his mother's body, his ear
against her heart, the child rediscovers the
familiar steady beat.
All is accomplished. All is perfect.
These two who have battled so fiercely are at
peace, at one again.

Maybe we can leave them alone together.
In fact, we should.
To remain would be an indiscretion.
Lovers should not be disturbed.
They don't want anyone to spoil the joy of
intimacy.
Since these two are true lovers, out of
respect and discretion, let us tiptoe from the
room, leaving them to share their new ecstasy.

As for us, we too have come a long way and learned
so much on the journey.
We were asking: If birth could be as painful, as cruel
for the child as it used to be for most mothers,
what is it that makes the experience so dreadful
for the child?
Now we know.
Since at last we have understood the message, understood
what the newborn is desperately trying to tell us with
his heartrending screams.
The message is very clear, and very simple indeed:
"I am in pain! I am suffering!"
But more than anything, "I AM AFRAID!"

2

Now we can see that fear and pain are one.
These children are echoing
what their mothers were, for so long, crying in labor.
Of course they never said it directly.
Who has the simplicity, the humility to say
"I am afraid!"?
Yet their poor bodies were nothing but a mass of
spasms, locked muscles, unbearable tensions, frantic
heavings that bore silent witness to their panic,
their terror.
What could they have been saying but "I am afraid, I am
terrified!"

By exorcising this fear, women have been freed from the agony of childbirth, and their experience transformed.

In the same way, by sparing the child this fear, this panic, we can transform birth into an enchantment.

3

Those who are skeptical or simply refuse to change things
might well say:
"All right. Quite possibly it's far from
pleasant to be born.
But what difference does it make?
It's all over in a few minutes. And afterward
who remembers? No one.
So then what does it matter how the child is received,
how he is welcomed?"
No one remembers?
Not only is that not true, but it is the complete opposite of
the truth.
The memory of birth and the terror that accompanies it
remains in each one of us.
But since it is so loaded with fear and pain, it
lies dormant and totally repressed, like a dreadful
secret at the bottom of our unconscious, like a
ship on the ocean floor.

But it is there, although we don't always know it.
Just like a name can be in our memory, but if it is
linked with unpleasant overtones, we think we can't
remember it.
Then again you might say if it is buried so deeply,
why dig it up, why not just let it rest?
Maybe we can't.
It is constantly trying to surface, and expresses itself
In our nightmares, our myths, our most
secret irrational inhibitions.
One could almost say that the root of all anguish
is an unconscious memory of birth and its
terrors.
Only those who have forgotten how it feels to wake up
at night, overwhelmed with panic, and the feeling that
lions and tigers were roaring under their bed,
ready to pounce, would deny the devastating
intensity of such fears, which are in fact nothing but
shadows of the original fear: the fear that is birth.

4

Fear.
How few of us are aware of how
much unconscious fear there is in our lives!
All this fear linked with the horror that is
birth.

One can only imagine what it would be like to be born

without this fear

or with this fear immediately extinguished like a fire

that's caught before it

gets a hold and becomes out of control.

Yes, if this fear could be extinguished before it can take

hold, how extraordinary life would be for one

so blessed.

The point of this book, of this whole story, is not just

to make birth something nice. It is far, far more

ambitious: it amounts to nothing less than a plan to give

birth to heroes, those extraordinary beings who seem free of

fear, and so can drink fully from the cup of life.

5

A plaguing question was why it seemed no one

was ever concerned about the child's plight, and even

ignored his anguish and despair.

Maybe there is something there that we ourselves do not

want to look at,

possibly because it might awaken something unpleasant

deep within ourselves that we'd rather not know about:

our own fear of death.

Strange, isn't it, that there seems to be such a deep
secret link between birth and death?
It is as if the fear of death, the dark shadow that casts
its gloom over our whole lives, is nothing but the
unconscious memory of . . . the fear we felt when
we were born.
So that . . . but then it's nearly too good to be true . . .
one born free of this fear would travel
through life as free as a bird.

6

Is this why we cut the cord in such a senseless, untimely
way?
Well, you might say, it's with the idea that it's going
to make the child breathe.
Why are we so anxious that he should breathe?
Of course there is the rational answer: lack of oxygen
will damage the brain—which is quite true.
But, as always, behind rationality is a deeper,
hidden reason.
Although no one is aware of it, those attending, watching
a baby being born, unconsciously, unknowingly
"hold their breath"!
As if finding themselves back at this terrible point, this
dramatic bridge between birth and death . . .

But because we do not have an umbilical cord beating for us, providing us with precious oxygen, the situation very quickly becomes unbearable . . . for us, that is to say.

"Do something! Do something!" clamors the unhappy voice within . . . the voice of our own anxiety.

While the easiest, most sensible thing for us to do would be to take a deep breath,

instead

we cut the cord!

The poor victim of this dramatic confusion, this unconscious projection, abruptly deprived of his umbilical cord and his previous supply of oxygen, suddenly finds himself choking to death.

In utter despair, he utters the abominable scream everyone was so anxiously expecting, which brings a smile to the faces of . . . the fools we are.

"Ah, he's breathing!" everyone exclaims with great relief.

"Ah, now *I* can breathe. I'm so relieved," is what we might say if we were just a little more clear and aware of what was going on . . . inside.

This process of projecting will now go on endlessly. And we proudly call it education.

But is birth really so important, one might ask.
It doesn't last long, you could say, compared with
what comes before and after it.
Maybe it's just a nasty moment to get through.
But that is perhaps somewhat glib. After all, there
is another "nasty moment" that, although equally brief,
nonetheless casts a long shadow, and that is death.
Yes, birth and the moments that follow, however few,
will leave a mark for the rest of life.
It is as if we are heading off in the wrong direction,
starting on the wrong foot.
It's like a boat leaving the harbor, with the poor captain
not knowing he has a faulty compass.
This compass, one might say, is
breathing.

7

When we are born we enter the kingdom of breath.
We embark on this endless oscillation that will carry us
through life to deliver us dutifully
into the hands of death.
Breath is the fragile vessel on which we cross this
ocean of life.
Everyone breathes, of course.
One could almost say that, in Nature, everything is breathing
continuously. Rhythmically.

But, for us, whether our breathing is free or impaired,
makes all the difference.

How many people go through life half-strangled, incapable
of a real sigh?

Much less a real laughter?

To live in freedom is to be able to breathe fully, freely.

Which requires a straight back.

That is to say, a spinal column that is free.

Free and supple, lithe, flexible.

And most people go through life with a broomstick for a
spine.

The mentally ill, for instance, are incapable of taking
a full deep breath.

If there is the least blockage along the spine, breathing—
which is the essence of life—is impaired.

The effects will be felt for a lifetime.

In the same way that no two people have the same face, no
two persons breathe in the same manner.

Everyone breathes his own way.

Usually very badly.

In fact, people say,

"I know I am not breathing well. Maybe I could learn."

Some people even try.

But maybe breathing is not something that can be learned.

The way we breathe was established, once and for all,
the moment we were born.

Far better to pay attention to it at that stage.

8

More dangerously, others will say: "Doubtless birth
does mark the child. But life is not a game. It's a
merciless battle. A jungle. So like it or not, you have to be
aggressive."
It is an error to imagine that birth without violence
produces children who are passive, weak, slow.
Quite the contrary.
Birth without violence produces children who are strong,
because they are free, without conflict.
Free and fully awake.
Aggression is not strength. It is the opposite.
Aggression and violence are the masks of weakness,
impotence, and fear.
Strength is sure, sovereign, and smiling.

But it would be hard to convince the advocates of violence
and aggression of this.
Because they have suffered themselves, their reaction is
to say:
"Life has been hard on me. I've been knocked around and
it's made me what I am. Let it be the same for my
children."
Which is as mean as saying:
"I've suffered. Let them suffer as well."
An eye for an eye.
The dreadful law of reprisal.

The vicious circle of action and reaction.
Leading only to endless misery and suffering.
Surely the best way to ensure that the bitter taste
will linger in our mouths forever.

You'll find it's the same people who say:
"So, women suffer in childbirth. It probably serves them
right."

9

What is it that makes these people so bitter, so angry?
They have not yet forgiven.
Unconsciously, they're still full of hatred for . . .
their own mothers.
It is this hatred that is at the root of all that
led us to the stake, the Inquisition, the Crusades.
All the abominable massacres committed in the name of
king and country, or even God.
This same hatred that is at the root of the feeling
of guilt, the feeling of sin.
Sin! There is no such thing as sin.
So-called sin is nothing but our own blindness and
ignorance.
Our forgetfulness of the panic that is birth for
the child.

As for pain and suffering, it satisfies no God.

If anyone doubts that in childbirth pain is unavoidable,

this new approach to birth proves the contrary.

10

What more can be said?

Only one thing.

Try.

Everything that has been said is so simple that one

feels embarrassed at having dwelled on it at such length.

Perhaps we have lost our taste for simplicity.

Once we've understood

the point of this whole story,

why don't we try?

Well, it takes . . . a lot of courage.

We also need patience and humility.

We must keep in mind that it is the child's first experience

of life.

As any good teacher knows, there is one sacred right:

the right of the child to experiment and make his own

discoveries.

Yes, patience, humility, and silence,

and the awareness that the newcomer is a person we meet

and greet after he has nearly drowned in a storm.

Oh, and of course . . .

Love.

Without love, the delivery room can be perfect, with the
right lighting, the walls soundproofed, the bath
temperature just right—and the child will
still scream.

If there is still any trace of nervousness, any suppressed
anger within ourselves, the baby will pick it up
immediately.

His judgment is frighteningly acute.

The baby knows everything. All in his own mysterious
way. He catches everything, sees right into our hearts,
knows the color of our thoughts, and all without language.

This is what is meant when the saint is likened to
the newborn.

Each sends us back our own image.

And so whenever a baby cries we must ask ourselves
the reason why.

11

"There's still something you haven't told us.
What becomes of these children born in silence?
Are they any different from other children?"
"It's something very subtle. You'd have to see for
yourself"
"All the same, can't you try to tell me?"
"We all go through life wearing masks. The mask of
tragedy far more often than the mask of comedy. And it is
this mask of tragedy that you see on the face of most
newborn babies:
their brows knitted and the corners of their little mouths
turned down.
A mask that hides their real faces and makes most of them
appear . . . ugly.

Their poor mothers are downcast, since they expected a 'lovely' baby.

Thank God, there is another mask.

A wide mouth lifted in a smile, with relaxed eyebrows and eyes crinkled with pleasure, not to say delight."

"But surely such a mask is never seen on a newborn baby?"

"You think not? Then why don't you look for yourself?"

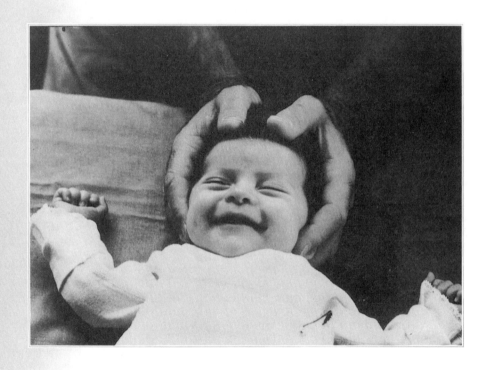

12

"Oh! This baby is really smiling. In fact he's in rapture!"

"It's hard to believe, isn't it?"

"But this picture hasn't got anything to do with what we've been discussing. The child you're showing me must be at least three months old.

Babies don't smile before that age."

"That's what people think. People and books.

As for the baby you see before you, he's not even twenty-four hours old."

"I . . . can't believe it."

"I must admit it's not the image of a newborn baby one is used to.

And yet there is still another mask."

"I'm not sure I follow you."

"You might say joy is not better than sorrow. It cannot last. Both are emotions that, after a while, cannot but turn into their opposite.

Laughter and tears are very close, you know.

Far better not to wear any mask. Far better to be free of emotions, both good and bad."

"Free . . . of emotions?

Whatever do you mean? I'm not sure I would like that.

And anyway, what's left for us if we don't have our emotions?"

"Well . . ."

Beyond
tears and laughter,
peace and serenity,
or
as they say in India,

Shanti! Shanti! Shanti!

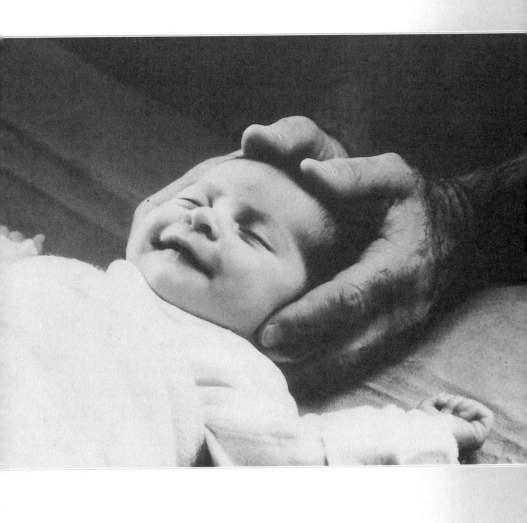

Afterword

Young women, this book has been written for you. So that you get back your courage. And take the great challenge. Childbirth is the Secret Garden of Women.

You have to protect it.

You'll have to make sure that no one enters it having in mind to rob you, to take away from you what is your most precious birthright, your greatest treasure: a fully conscious, enlightened delivery.

Birth without Violence is telling a story. Stories are very important. As important as dreams. Without which, as we all know, life becomes impossible.

A story. A love story. The one love story behind all love stories. *Birth without Violence* is a literary text, a book of poetry. So allow me to conclude with one more touch of poetry.

As a farewell.

As a blessing, as well.

Divine Water, Almighty Sea
all life is born
out of thee
only to
die

and who am I to
ask you
why!

all life and
I must
die

at times you're very hard
and yet I know that
you love me

far more, far more
than I can ever
thank you
for

therefore to Thee I'll bow
with love and
awe

Divine Water, All Mighty Sea
Divine Mother, Almighty

Thee

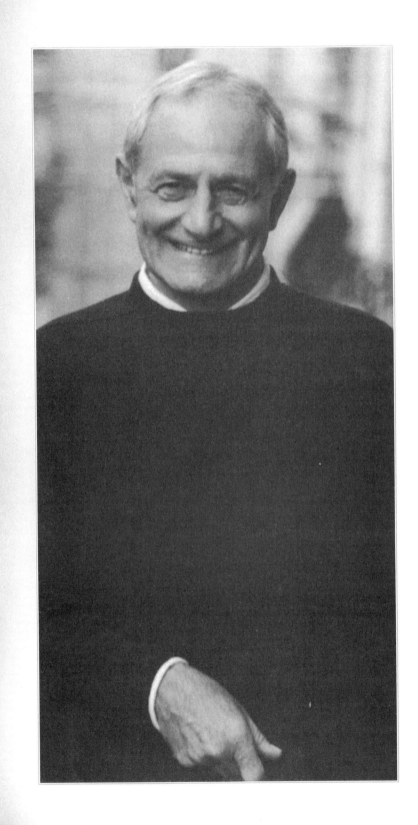

About the Author

Born in France in 1918, Frédérick Leboyer graduated from the University of Paris School of Medicine, where he became Chef de Clinique in the 1950s. During his time as an obstetrician, he attended more than ten thousand births. He became increasingly dissatisfied with the impersonal clinical treatment of the newborn child and began working on new ideas about the process of birth. This reassessment resulted in the groundbreaking *Birth without Violence*, first published in France in 1974. This book revolutionized the course of prenatal care and the way babies are introduced into the world, and with this edition will continue to gently welcome a new generation of infants.

Frédérick Leboyer first visited India in 1959 and spent two months a year there in the following two decades. He developed a deep interest in yoga and its applications to pregnancy and childbirth, especially in the use of breathing and sound.

Three years after the publication of *Birth without Violence*, Leboyer wrote *Loving Hands*, a book inspired by his observation in Calcutta of a young mother named Shantala lovingly massaging her baby. In her honor, Leboyer gave her name to this form of massage. He has also published *Inner Beauty, Inner Light* in 1978, *The Art of Breathing* in 1991, and *The Art of Giving Birth*, a translation of *Atmen, singen, gebären* [Breathing, Singing, Giving Birth] in 2009.

Frédérick Leboyer is credited as the founder of the modern gentle birth movement. Since his retirement, Leboyer has conducted seminars and workshops all over the world for pregnant women, midwives, gynecologists, and pediatricians. He lives in Switzerland.